The Complete Keto Chaffle Cooking Guide

Get in Shape and Lose Weight with Tasty and Affordable Recipes for Beginners

Kade Harrison

Table of Contents

Cream Cake Chaffle

Servings: 4

Cooking Time:

12 Minutes

Ingredients:

- Chaffle
- 4 oz cream cheese, softened
- 4 eggs
- 4 tbsp coconut flour
- 1 tbsp almond flour
- 1 ½ tsp baking powder
- 1 tbsp butter, softened
- 1 tsp vanilla extract
- ½ tsp cinnamon
- 1 tbsp sweetener
- 1 tbsp shredded coconut, colored and unsweetened
- 1 tbsp walnuts, chopped
- Italian Cream Frosting
- 2 oz cream cheese, softened
- 2 tbsp butter, room temperature
- 2 tbsp sweetener
- ½ tsp vanilla

Directions:

1. Preheat your waffle maker and add ¼ of the
2. Cook for 3 minutes and repeat the process until you have 4 chaffles.
3. Remove and set aside.
4. In the meantime, start making your frosting by mixing all the

5. Stir until you have a smooth and creamy mixture.
6. Cool, frost the cake and enjoy.

Nutrition:

Calories per Servings: 127 Kcal ; Fats: 10 g ; Carbs: 5.5 g ; Protein: 7 g

Almond Butter Chaffles

Servings: 2

Cooking Time:

10 Minutes

Ingredients:

- 1 large organic egg, beaten
- 1/3 cup Mozzarella cheese, shredded
- 1 tablespoon Erythritol
- 2 tablespoons almond butter
- 1 teaspoon organic vanilla extract

Directions:

1. Preheat a mini waffle iron and then grease it.
2. In a medium bowl, place all ingredients and with a fork, mix until well combined.
3. Place half of the mixture into preheated waffle iron and cook for about 5 minutes or until golden brown.
4. Repeat with the remaining mixture.
5. Serve warm.

Nutrition:

Calories: 153 Net Carb: 2 g Fat: 12.3 g Saturated Fat: 2 g Carbohydrates: 3 Dietary Fiber: 1.6 g Sugar: 1.2 g Protein: 7.9 g

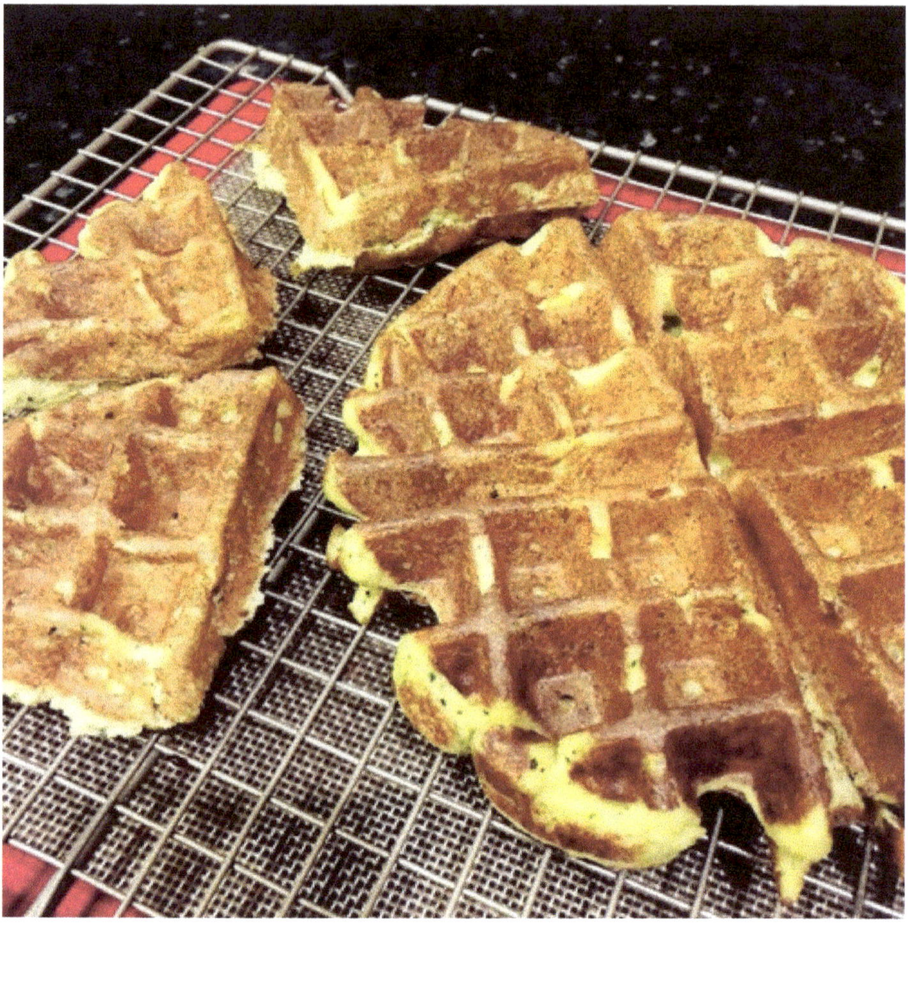

Layered Chaffles

Servings: 2

Cooking Time:

10 Minutes

Ingredients:

- 1 organic egg, beaten and divided
- ½ cup cheddar cheese, shredded and divided
- Pinch of salt

Directions:

1. Preheat a mini waffle iron and then grease it.
2. Place about 1/8 cup of cheese in the bottom of the waffle iron and top with half of the beaten egg.
3. Now, place 1/8 cup of cheese on top and cook for about 4–5 minutes.
4. Repeat with the remaining cheese and egg.
5. Serve warm.

Nutrition:

Calories 145 Net Carbs 0.5 g Total Fat 11.g Saturated Fat 6.6 g Cholesterol 112 mg Sodium 284 g Total Carbs 0.5 g Fiber 0 g Sugar 0.3 g Protein 9.8 g

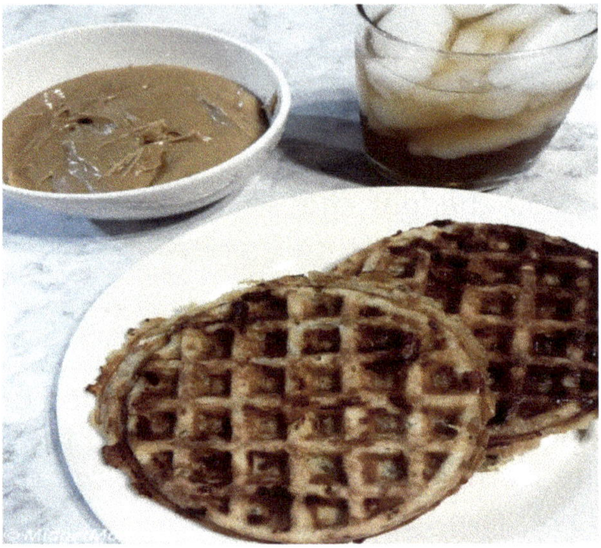

Simple Mozzarella Chaffles

Servings: 2

Cooking Time:

8 Minutes

Ingredients:

- ½ cup mozzarella cheese, shredded
- 1 large organic egg
- 2 tablespoons blanched almond flour
- ¼ teaspoon organic baking powder
- 2–3 drops liquid stevia

Directions:

1. Preheat a mini waffle iron and then grease it.
2. In a medium bowl, put all ingredients and with a fork, mix until well combined.Place half of the mixture into preheated waffle iron and cook for about 3–4 minutes.
3. Repeat with the remaining mixture.
4. Serve warm.

Nutrition:

Calories 98 Net Carbs 1.4 g Total Fat 7.1 g Saturated Fat 1.8 g Cholesterol 97 mg Sodium 81 mg Total Carbs 2.2 g Fiber 0.8 g Sugar 0.2 g Protein 6.7 g

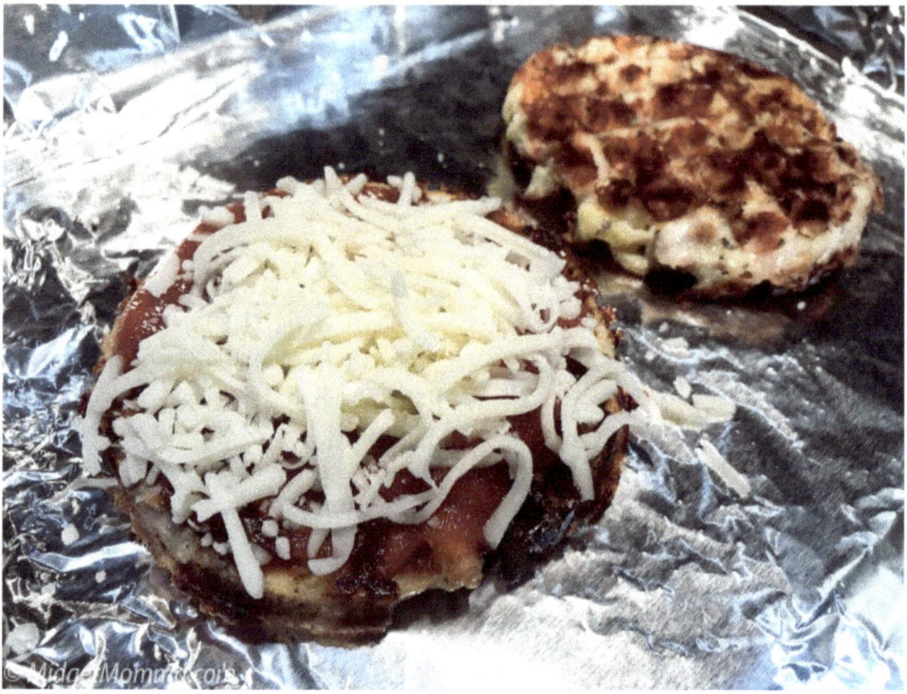

Cream Mini-chaffles

Servings: 2

Cooking Time:

10 Minutes

Ingredients:

- 2 tsp coconut flour
- 4 tsp swerve/monk fruit
- ¼ tsp baking powder
- 1 egg
- 1 oz cream cheese
- ½ tsp vanilla extract

Directions:

1. Turn on waffle maker to heat and oil it with cooking spray.
2. Mix swerve/monk fruit, coconut flour, and baking powder in a small mixing bowl.
3. Add cream cheese, egg, vanilla extract, and whisk until well-combined.
4. Add batter into waffle maker and cook for 3-minutes, until golden brown.
5. Serve with your favorite toppings.

Nutrition:

Carbs: 4 g ; Fat: g ;Protein: 2 g ;Calories: 73

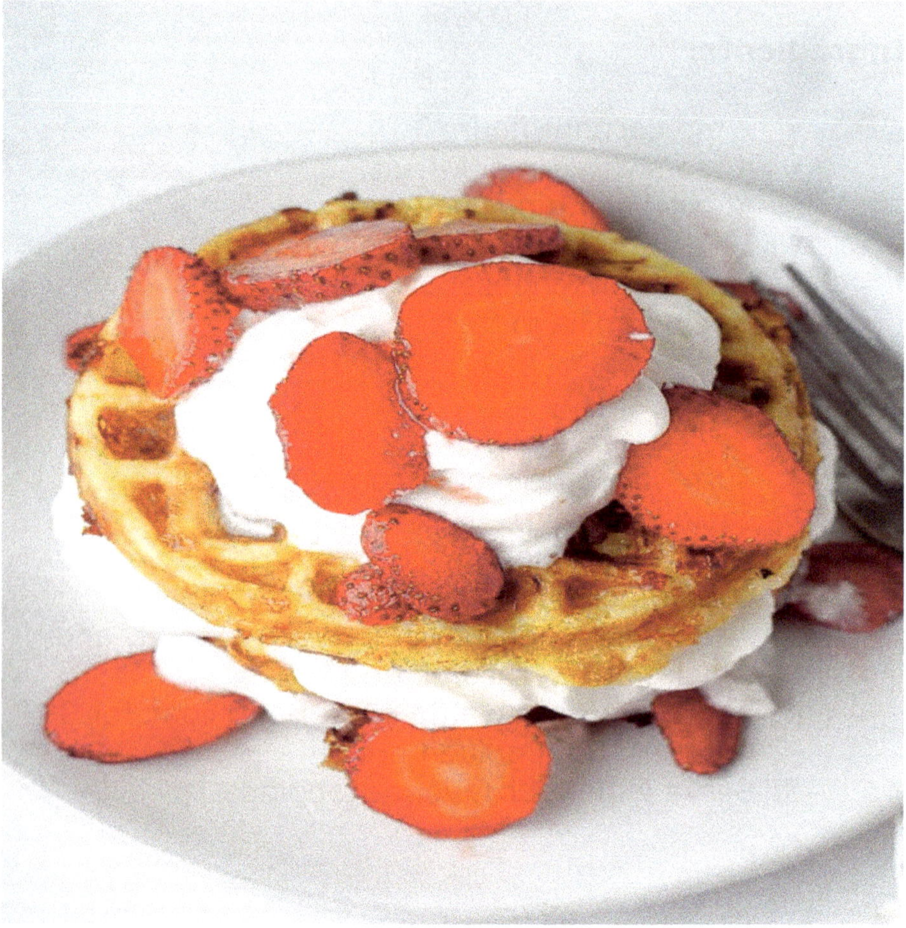

Raspberry Chaffles

Servings: 2

Cooking Time:

5 Minutes

Ingredients:

- 4 Tbsp almond flour
- 4 large eggs
- 2⅓ cup shredded mozzarella cheese
- 1 tsp vanilla extract
- 1 Tbsp erythritol sweetener
- 1½ tsp baking powder
- ½ cup raspberries

Directions:

1. Turn on waffle maker to heat and oil it with cooking spray.
2. Mix almond flour, sweetener, and baking powder in a bowl.
3. Add cheese, eggs, and vanilla extract, and mix until well-combined.
4. Add 1 portion of batter to waffle maker and spread it evenly. Close and cook for 3-minutes, or until golden.
5. Repeat until remaining batter is used.
6. Serve with raspberries.

Nutrition:

Carbs: 5 g ;Fat: 11 g ;Protein: 24 g ;Calories: 300

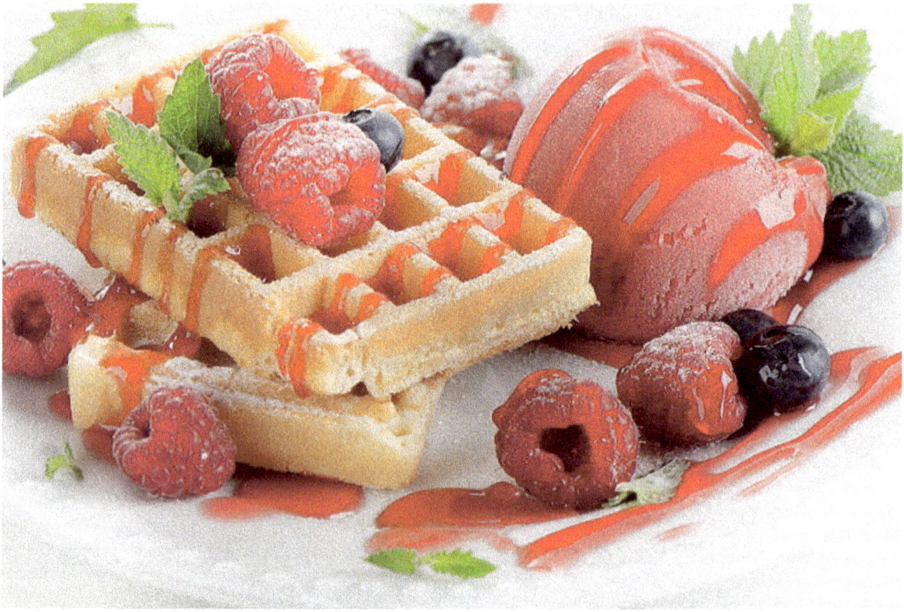

Lemon Chaffles

Servings: 2

Cooking Time:

10 Minutes

Ingredients:

- 1 organic egg, beaten
- 1 ounce cream cheese, softened
- 2 tablespoons almond flour
- 1 tablespoon fresh lemon juice
- 2 teaspoons Erythritol
- ½ teaspoon fresh lemon zest, grated
- ¼ teaspoon organic baking powder
- Pinch of salt
- ½ teaspoon powdered Erythritol

Directions:

1. Preheat a mini waffle iron and then grease it.
2. In a bowl, place all ingredients except the powdered Erythritol and beat until well combined.
3. Place half of the mixture into preheated waffle iron and cook for about 5 minutes or until golden brown.
4. Repeat with the remaining mixture.
5. Serve warm with the sprinkling of powdered Erythritol.

Nutrition:

Calories: 129 Net Carb: 1.2 g Fat: 10.9 g Saturated Fat: 4.1 g Carbohydrates: 2.4 g Dietary Fiber: 0.8 g Sugar: 0. Protein: 3.9 g

Chocolate Chip Chaffles

Servings: 1

Cooking Time:

6 Minutes

Ingredients:

- 1 egg
- 1 tsp coconut flour
- 1 tsp sweetener
- ½ tsp vanilla extract
- ¼ cup heavy whipping cream, for serving
- ½ cup almond milk ricotta, finely shredded
- 2 tbsp sugar-free chocolate chips

Directions:

1. Preheat your mini waffle iron.
2. Mix the egg, coconut flour, vanilla, and sweetener. Whisk together with a fork.
3. Stir in the almond milk ricotta.
4. Pour half of the batter into the waffle iron and dot with a pinch of chocolate chips.
5. Close the waffle iron and cook for minutes.
6. Repeat with remaining batter.
7. Serve hot with the whipped cream.

Nutrition:

Calories per Servings: 304 Kcal ; Fats: 16 g ; Carbs: 7 g ; Protein: 3 g

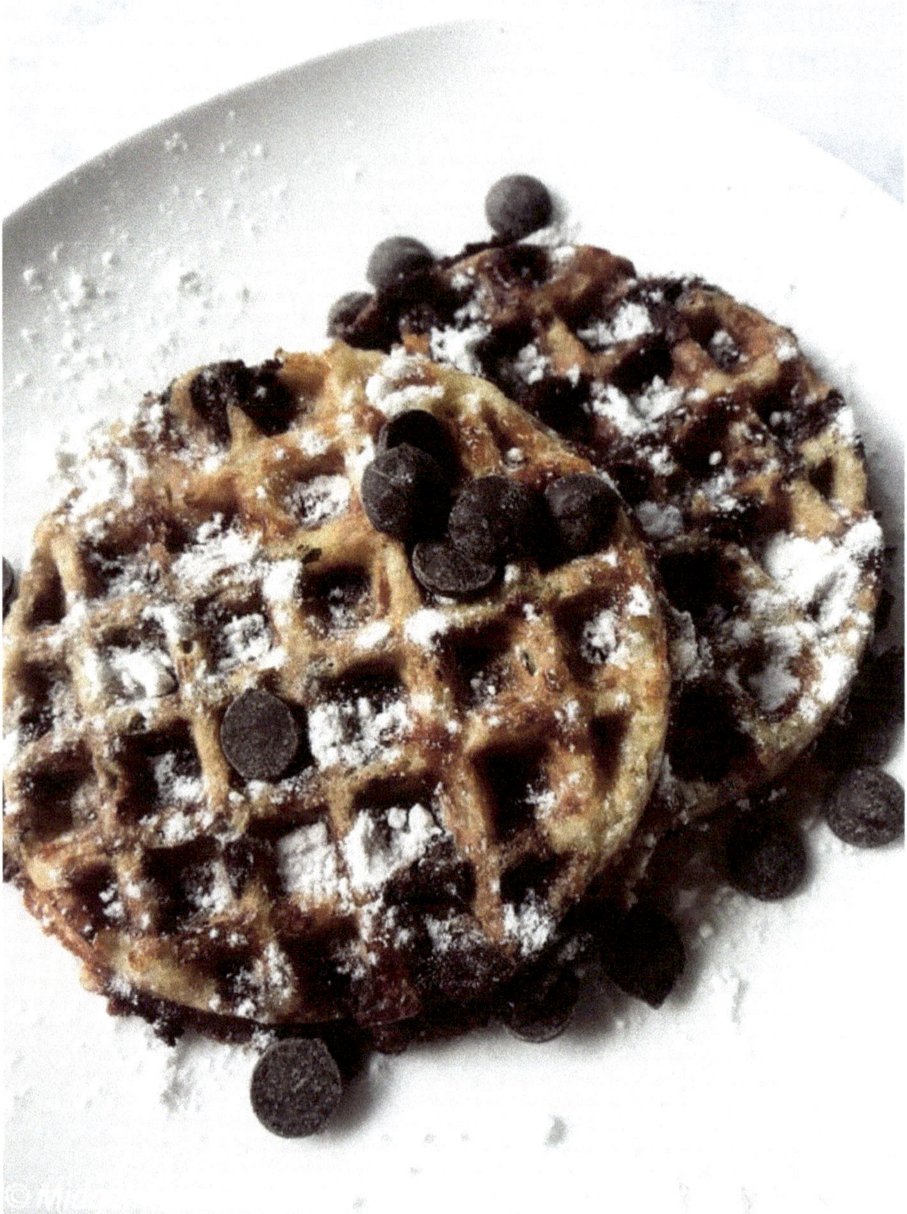

Pumpkin & Psyllium Husk Chaffles

Servings: 4

Cooking Time:

16 Minutes

Ingredients:

- 2 organic eggs
- ½ cup mozzarella cheese, shredded
- 1 tablespoon homemade pumpkin puree
- 2 teaspoons Erythritol
- ½ teaspoon psyllium husk powder
- 1/3 teaspoon ground cinnamon
- Pinch of salt
- ½ teaspoon organic vanilla extract

Directions:

1. Preheat a mini waffle iron and then grease it.
2. In a bowl, place all ingredients and beat until well combined.
3. Place ¼ of the mixture into preheated waffle iron and cook for about 4 minutes or until golden brown.
4. Repeat with the remaining mixture.
5. Serve warm.

Nutrition:

Calories: 4 Carb: 0.6 g Fat: 2.8 g Saturated Fat: 1.1 g Carbohydrates: 0.8 g Dietary Fiber: 0.2 g Sugar: 0.4 g Protein: 3.9 g

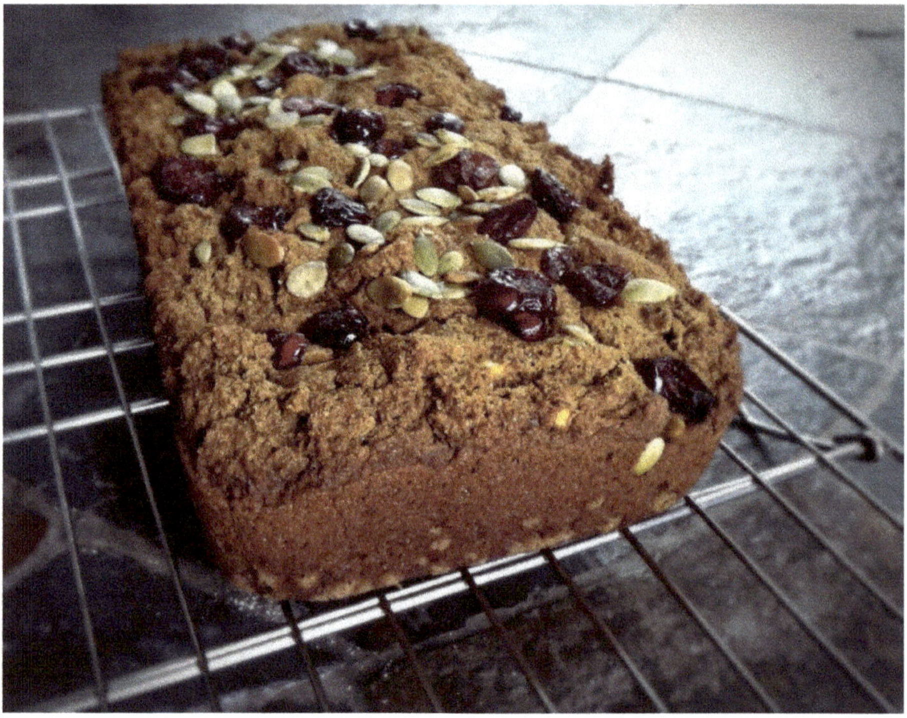

Blackberry Chaffles

Servings: 2

Cooking Time:

8 Minutes

Ingredients:

- 1 organic egg, beaten
- 1/3 cup Mozzarella cheese, shredded
- 1 teaspoon cream cheese, softened
- 1 teaspoon coconut flour
- ¼ teaspoon organic baking powder
- ¾ teaspoon powdered Erythritol
- ¼ teaspoon ground cinnamon
- ¼ teaspoon organic vanilla extract
- Pinch of salt
- 1 tablespoon fresh blackberries

Directions:

1. Preheat a mini waffle iron and then grease it.
2. In a bowl, place all ingredients except for blackberries and beat until well combined.
3. Fold in the blackberries.
4. Place half of the mixture into preheated waffle iron and cook for about minutes or until golden brown.
5. Repeat with the remaining mixture.
6. Serve warm.

Nutrition:

Calories: 121 Net Carb: 2 Fat: 7.5 g Saturated Fat: 3.3 g Carbohydrates: 4.5 g Dietary Fiber: 1.8 g Sugar: 0.9 g Protein: 8.9 g

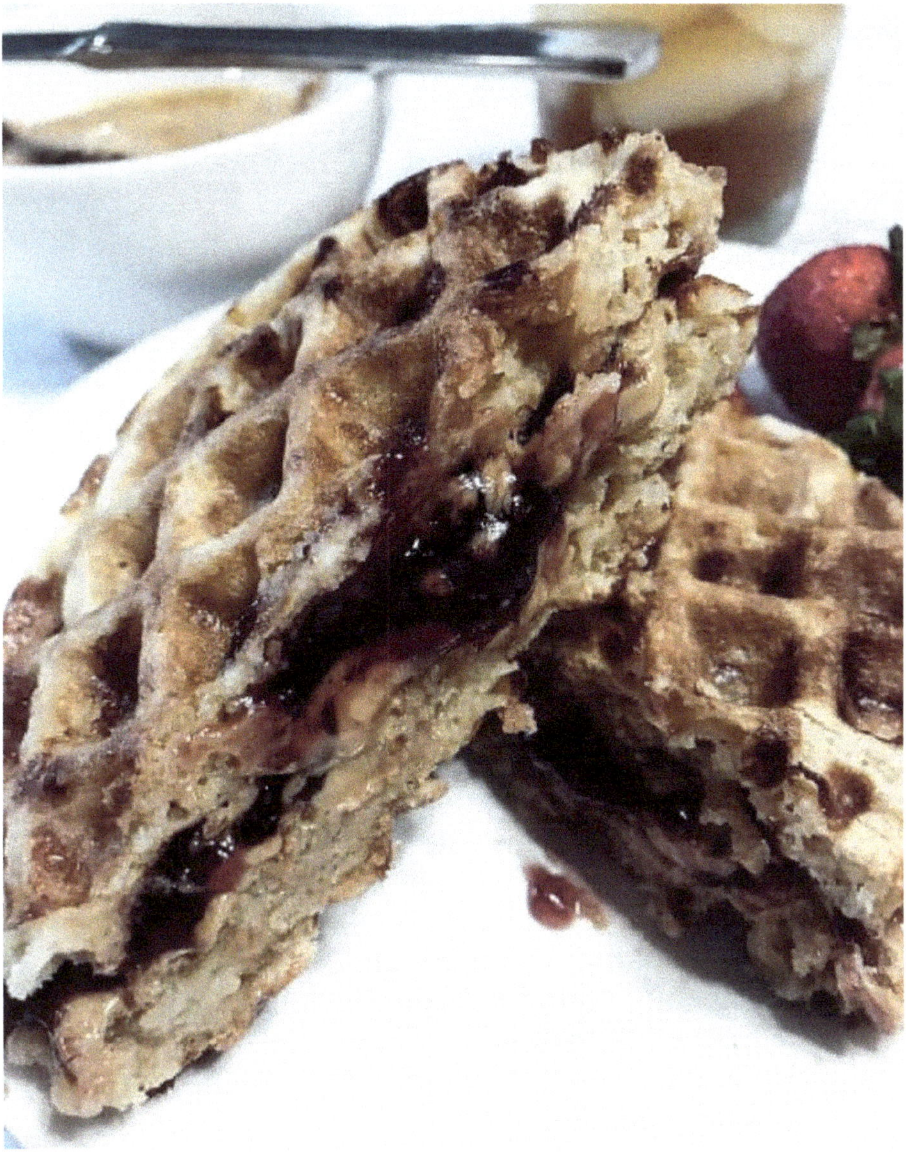

Pumpkin Cream Cheese Chaffles

Servings: 2

Cooking Time:

10 Minutes

Ingredients:

- 1 organic egg, beaten
- ½ cup Mozzarella cheese, shredded
- 1½ tablespoon sugar-free pumpkin puree
- 2 teaspoons heavy cream
- 1 teaspoon cream cheese, softened
- 1 tablespoon almond flour
- 1 tablespoon Erythritol
- ½ teaspoon pumpkin pie spice
- ½ teaspoon organic baking powder
- 1 teaspoon organic vanilla extract

Directions:

1. Preheat a mini waffle iron and then grease it.
2. In a medium bowl, place all ingredients and with a fork, mix until well combined.
3. Place half of the mixture into preheated waffle iron and cook for about 5 minutes or until golden brown.
4. Repeat with the remaining mixture.
5. Serve warm.

Nutrition:

Calories: 110 Net Carb: 2.5 g Fat: 4.3 g Saturated Fat: 1 g Carbohydrates: 3.3 g Dietary Fiber: 0.8 g Sugar: 1 g Protein: 5.2 g

Cinnamon Pecan Chaffles

Servings: 1

Cooking Time:

40 Minutes

Ingredients:

- 1 Tbsp butter
- 1 egg
- ½ tsp vanilla
- 2 Tbsp almond flour
- 1 Tbsp coconut flour
- ⅛ tsp baking powder
- 1 Tbsp monk fruit
- For the crumble:
- ½ tsp cinnamon
- 1 Tbsp melted butter
- 1 tsp monk fruit
- 1 Tbsp chopped pecans

Directions:

1. Turn on waffle maker to heat and oil it with cooking spray.
2. Melt butter in a bowl, then mix in the egg and vanilla.
3. Mix in remaining chaffle ingredients.
4. Combine crumble ingredients in a separate bowl.
5. Pour half of the chaffle mix into waffle maker. Top with half of crumble mixture.
6. Cook for 5 minutes, or until done.
7. Repeat with the other half of the batter.

Nutrition:

Carbs: g ;Fat: 35 g ;Protein: 10 g ;Calories: 391

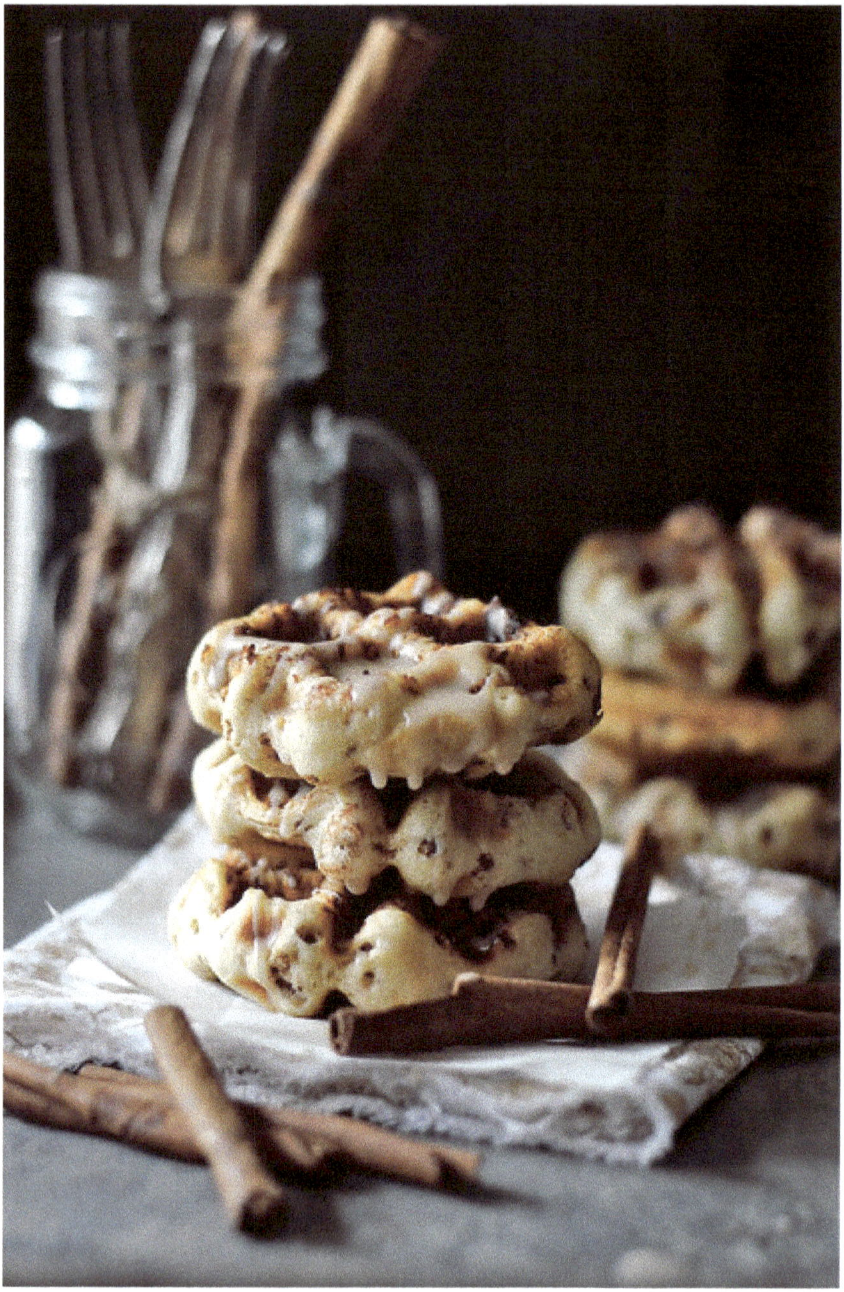

Chaffle Glazed With Raspberry

Servings: 1

Cooking Time:

5 Minutes

Ingredients:

- Donut Chaffle Ingredients:
- 1 egg
- ¼ cup mozzarella cheese, shredded
- 2 tsp cream cheese, softened
- 1 tsp sweetener
- 1tsp almond flour
- ½ tsp baking powder
- 20 drops glazed donut flavoring
- Raspberry Jelly Filling:
- ¼ cup raspberries
- 1 tsp chia seeds
- 1 tsp confectioners sweetener
- Donut Glaze:
- 1 tsp powdered sweetener
- Heavy whipping cream

Directions:

1. Spray your waffle maker with cooking oil and add the batter mixture into the waffle maker.
2. Cook for 3 minutes and set aside.
3. Raspberry Jelly Filling:
4. Mix all the
5. Place in a pot and heat on medium.
6. Gently mash the raspberries and set aside to cool. Donut Glaze:
7. Stir together the
8. Assembling:

9. Lay your chaffles on a plate and add the fillings mixture between the layers.
10. Drizzle the glaze on top and enjoy.

Nutrition:

Calories per Servings: 188 Kcal ; Fats: 23 g ; Carbs: 12 g ; Protein: 17 g

Oreo Keto Chaffles

Servings: 2

Cooking Time:

5 Minutes

Ingredients:

- 1 egg
- 1½ Tbsp unsweetened cocoa
- 2 Tbsp lakanto monk fruit, or choice of sweetener
- 1 Tbsp heavy cream
- 1 tsp coconut flour
- ½ tsp baking powder
- ½ tsp vanilla
- For the cheese cream:
- 1 Tbsp lakanto powdered sweetener
- 2 Tbsp softened cream cheese
- ¼ tsp vanilla

Directions:

1. Turn on waffle maker to heat and oil it with cooking spray.
2. Combine all chaffle ingredients in a small bowl.
3. Pour one half of the chaffle mixture into waffle maker. Cook for 5 minutes.
4. Remove and repeat with the second half if the mixture. Let chaffles sit for 2-3 to crisp up.
5. Combine all cream ingredients and spread on chaffle when they have cooled to room temperature.

Nutrition:

Carbs: 3 g ;Fat: 4 g ;Protein: 7 g ;Calories:

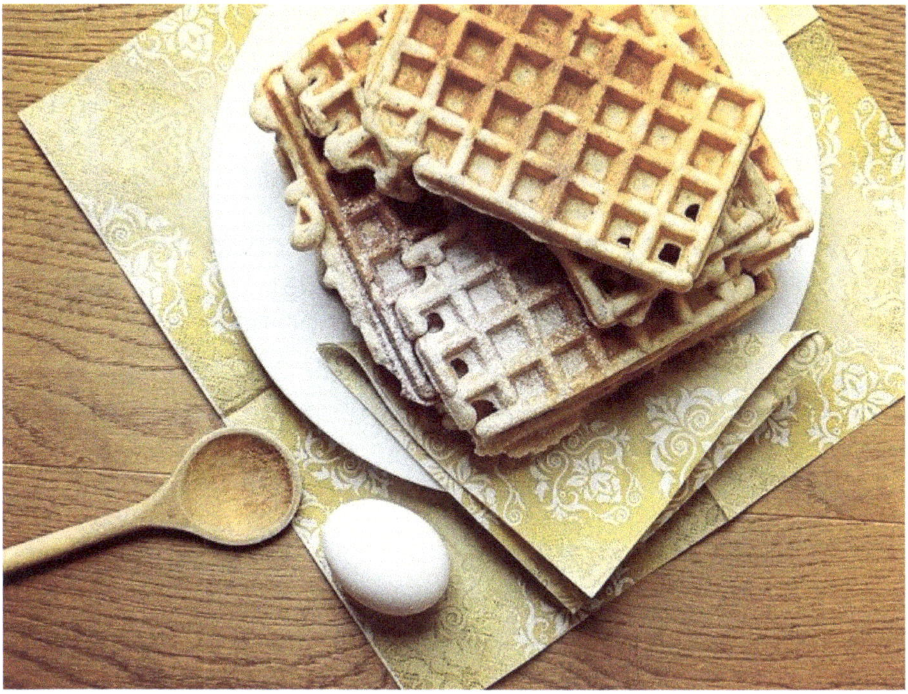

Cinnamon Sugar Chaffles

Servings: 2

Cooking Time:

12 Minutes

Ingredients:

- 2 eggs
- 1 cup Mozzarella cheese, shredded
- 2 tbsp blanched almond flour
- ½ tbsp butter, melted
- 2 tbsp Erythritol
- ½ tsp cinnamon
- ½ tsp vanilla extract
- ½ tsp psyllium husk powder, optional
- ¼ tsp baking powder, optional
- 1 tbsp melted butter, for topping
- ¼ cup Erythritol, for topping
- ¾ tsp cinnamon, for topping

Directions:

1. Pour enough batter into the waffle maker and cook for 4 minutes.
2. Once the cooked, carefully remove the chaffle and set aside.
3. Repeat with the remaining batter the same steps.
4. Stir together the cinnamon and erythritol.
5. Finish by brushing your chaffles with the melted butter and then sprinkle with cinnamon sugar.

Nutrition:

Calories: 208 Kcal ; Fats: 16 g ; Carbs: 4 g ; Protein: 11 g

Cream Cheese Chaffles

Servings: 2

Cooking Time:

8 Minutes

Ingredients:

- 2 teaspoons coconut flour
- 3 teaspoons Erythritol
- ¼ teaspoon organic baking powder
- 1 organic egg, beaten
- 1 ounce cream cheese, softened
- ½ teaspoon organic vanilla extract

Directions:

6. Preheat a mini waffle iron and then grease it.
7. In a bowl, place flour, Erythritol and baking powder and mix well.
8. Add the egg, cream cheese and vanilla extract and beat until well combined.
9. Place half of the mixture into preheated waffle iron and cook for about 3-minutes or until golden brown.
10. Repeat with the remaining mixture.
11. Serve warm.

Nutrition:

Calories: 95 Net Carb: 1.6 g Fat: 4 g Saturated Fat: 4 g Carbohydrates: 2.6 g Dietary Fiber: 1 g Sugar: 0.3 g Protein: 4.2 g

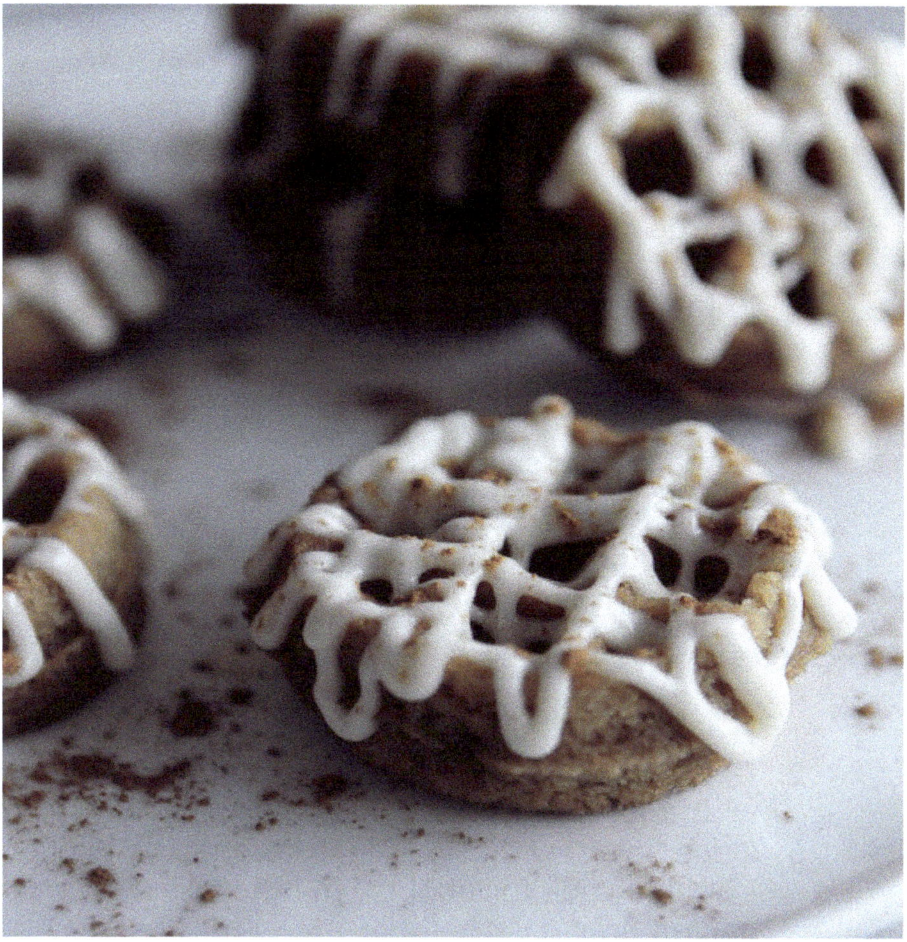

Mozzarella & Butter Chaffles

Servings: 2

Cooking Time:

8 Minutes

Ingredients:

- 1 large organic egg, beaten
- ¾ cup Mozzarella cheese, shredded
- ½ tablespoon unsalted butter, melted
- 2 tablespoons blanched almond flour
- 2 tablespoons Erythritol
- ½ teaspoon ground cinnamon
- ½ teaspoon Psyllium husk powder
- ¼ teaspoon organic baking powder
- ½ teaspoon organic vanilla extract

Directions:

1. Preheat a waffle iron and then grease it.
2. In a medium bowl, place all ingredients and with a fork, mix until well combined.
3. Place half of the mixture into preheated waffle iron and cook for about 5 minutes or until golden brown.
4. Repeat with the remaining mixture.
5. Serve warm.

Nutrition:

Calories: 140 Net Carb: 1.9 g Fat: 10 Saturated Fat: 4 g Carbohydrates: 3 g Dietary Fiber: 1.1 g Sugar: 0.3 g Protein: 7.8 g

Pumpkin Pecan Chaffles

Servings: 2

Cooking Time:

10 Minutes

Ingredients:

- 1 egg
- ½ cup mozzarella cheese grated
- 1 Tbsp pumpkin puree
- ½ tsp pumpkin spice
- 1 tsp erythritol low carb sweetener
- 2 Tbsp almond flour
- 2 Tbsp pecans, toasted chopped
- 1 cup heavy whipped cream
- ¼ cup low carb caramel sauce

Directions:

1. Turn on waffle maker to heat and oil it with cooking spray.
2. In a bowl, beat egg.
3. Mix in mozzarella, pumpkin, flour, pumpkin spice, and erythritol.
4. Stir in pecan pieces.
5. Spoon one half of the batter into waffle maker and spread evenly.
6. Close and cook for 5 minutes.
7. Remove cooked waffles to a plate.
8. Repeat with remaining batter.
9. Serve with pecans, whipped cream, and low carb caramel sauce.

Nutrition:

Carbs: 4 g ; Fat: 17 g ;Protein: 11 g ;Calories: 210

Chocolate Cream Chaffles

Servings: 2

Cooking Time:

10 Minutes

Ingredients:

- 1 organic egg
- 1½ tablespoons cacao powder
- 2 tablespoons Erythritol
- 1 tablespoon heavy cream
- 1 teaspoon coconut flour
- ½ teaspoon organic baking powder
- ½ teaspoon organic vanilla extract
- ½ teaspoon powdered Erythritol

Directions:

1. Preheat a mini waffle iron and then grease it.
2. In a bowl, place all ingredients except the powdered Erythritol and beat until well combined.
3. Place half of the mixture into preheated waffle iron and cook for about 5 minutes or until golden brown.
4. Repeat with the remaining mixture.
5. Serve warm with the sprinkling of powdered Erythritol.

Nutrition:

Calories: 7 Carb: 2.1 g Fat: 5.9 g Saturated Fat: 3 g Carbohydrates: 3.8 g Dietary Fiber: 1.7 g Sugar: 0.3 g Protein: 3.8 g

Blueberry Cinnamon Chaffles

Servings: 3

Cooking Time:

10 Minutes

Ingredients:

- 1 cup shredded mozzarella cheese
- 3 Tbsp almond flour
- 2 eggs
- 2 tsp Swerve or granulated sweetener of choice
- 1 tsp cinnamon
- ½ tsp baking powder
- ½ cup fresh blueberries
- ½ tsp of powdered Swerve

Directions:

1. Turn on waffle maker to heat and oil it with cooking spray.
2. Mix eggs, flour, mozzarella, cinnamon, vanilla extract, sweetener, and baking powder in a bowl until well combined.
3. Add in blueberries.
4. Pour ¼ batter into each waffle mold.
5. Close and cook for 8 minutes.
6. If it's crispy and the waffle maker opens without pulling the chaffles apart, the chaffle is ready. If not, close and cook for 1-2 minutes more.
7. Serve with favorite topping and more blueberries.

Nutrition:

Carbs: 9 g ; Fat: 12 g ; Protein: 13 g ;Calories: 193

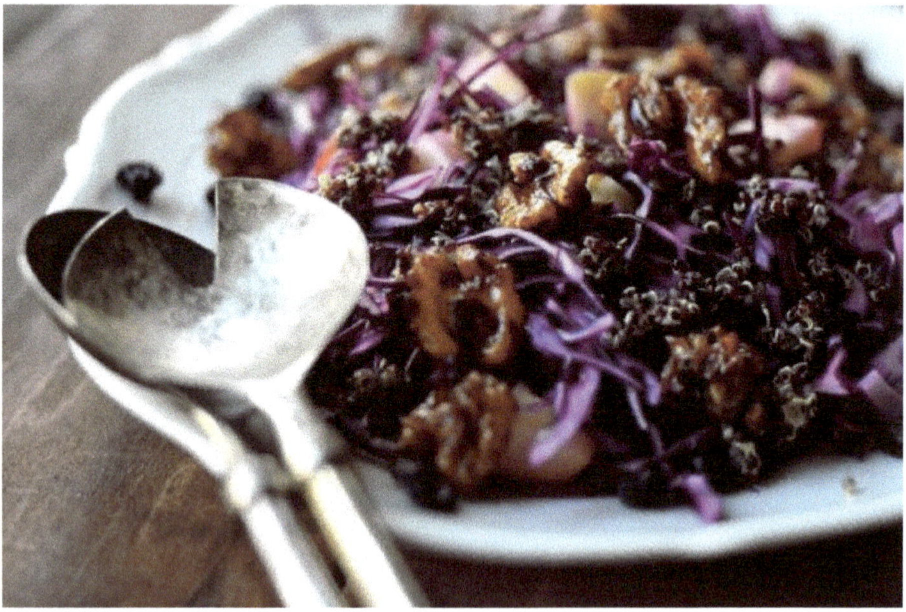

Gingerbread Chaffle

Servings: 2

Cooking Time:

5 Minutes

Ingredients:

- ½ cup mozzarella cheese grated
- 1 medium egg
- ½ tsp baking powder
- 1 tsp erythritol powdered
- ½ tsp ground ginger
- ¼ tsp ground nutmeg
- ½ tsp ground cinnamon
- ⅛ tsp ground cloves
- 2 Tbsp almond flour
- 1 cup heavy whipped cream
- ¼ cup keto-friendly maple syrup

Directions:

1. Turn on waffle maker to heat and oil it with cooking spray.
2. Beat egg in a bowl.
3. Add flour, mozzarella, spices, baking powder, and erythritol. Mix well.
4. Spoon one half of the batter into waffle maker and spread out evenly.
5. Close and cook for minutes.
6. Remove cooked chaffle and repeat with remaining batter.
7. Serve with whipped cream and maple syrup.

Nutrition:

Carbs: 5 g; Fat: 15 g; Protein: 12 g; Calories: 103

Chocolate Whipping Cream Chaffles

Servings: 2

Cooking Time:

8 Minutes

Ingredients:

- 1 tablespoon almond flour
- 2 tablespoons cacao powder
- 2 tablespoons granulated Erythritol
- ¼ teaspoon organic baking powder
- 1 organic egg
- 1 tablespoon heavy whipping cream
- ¼ teaspoon organic vanilla extract
- 1/8 teaspoon organic almond extract

Directions:

1. Preheat a mini waffle iron and then grease it.
2. In a bowl, place all ingredients and beat until well combined.
3. Place half of the mixture into preheated waffle iron and cook for about 4 minutes or until golden brown.
4. Repeat with the remaining mixture.
5. Serve warm.

Nutrition:

Calories: 94 Net Carb: 2 g Fat: 7.9 g Saturated Fat: 3.2 g Carbohydrates: 3.9 g Dietary Fiber: 1.9 g Sugar: 0.4 g Protein: 3.9 g

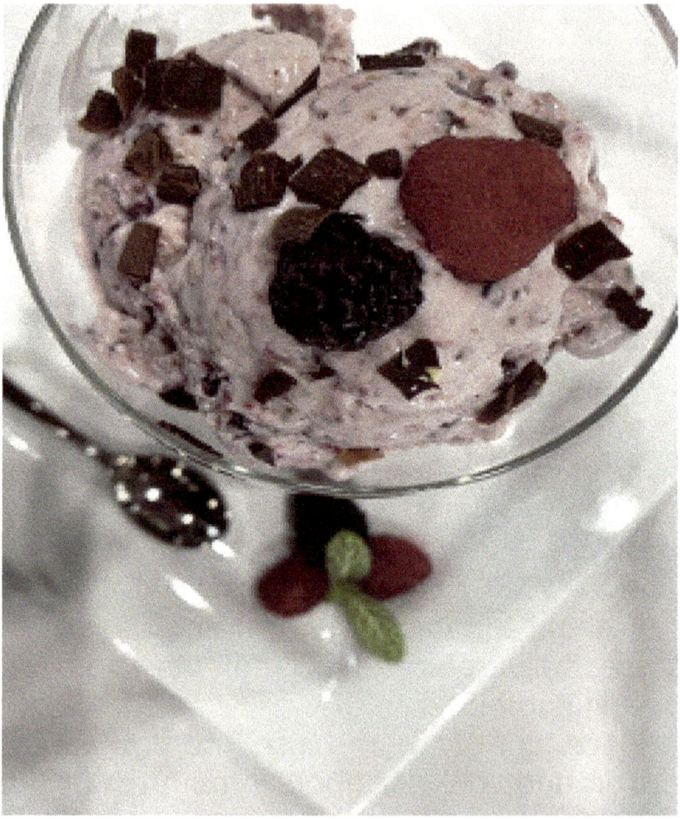

Almond Flour Chaffles

Servings: 2

Cooking Time:

20 Minutes

Ingredients:

- 1 large egg
- 1 Tbsp blanched almond flour
- ¼ tsp baking powder
- ½ cup shredded mozzarella cheese

Directions:

1. Whisk egg, almond flour, and baking powder together.
2. Stir in mozzarella and set batter aside.
3. Turn on waffle maker to heat and oil it with cooking spray.
4. Pour half of the batter onto waffle maker and spread it evenly with a spoon.
5. Cook for 3 minutes, or until it reaches desired doneness.
6. Transfer to a plate and repeat with remaining batter.
7. Let chaffles cool for 2-3 minutes to crisp up.

Nutrition:

Carbs: 2 g ;Fat: 13 g ;Protein: 10 g ;Calories: 131

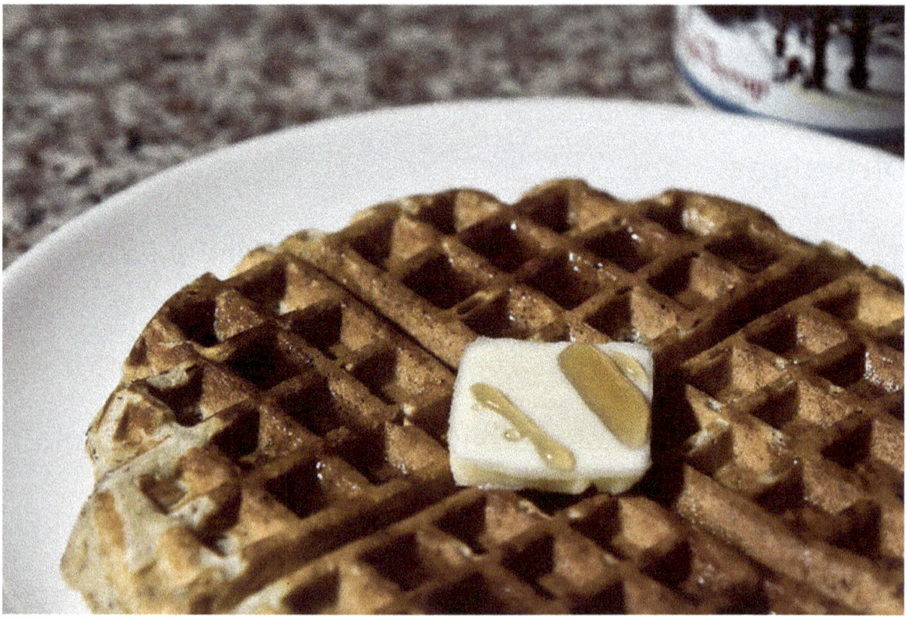

Strawberry Shortcake Chaffles

Servings: 1

Cooking Time:

25 Minutes

Ingredients:

- For the batter:
- 1 egg
- ¼ cup mozzarella cheese
- 1 Tbsp cream cheese
- ¼ tsp baking powder
- 2 strawberries, sliced
- 1 tsp strawberry extract
- For the glaze:
- 1 Tbsp cream cheese
- ¼ tsp strawberry extract
- 1 Tbsp monk fruit confectioners blend
- For the whipped cream:
- 1 cup heavy whipping cream
- 1 tsp vanilla
- 1 Tbsp monk fruit

Directions:

1. Turn on waffle maker to heat and oil it with cooking spray.
2. Beat egg in a small bowl.
3. Add remaining batter components.
4. Divide the mixture in half.
5. Cook one half of the batter in a waffle maker for 4 minutes, or until golden brown.
6. Repeat with remaining batter
7. Mix all glaze ingredients and spread over each warm chaffle.

8. Mix all whipped cream ingredients and whip until it starts to form peaks.
9. Top each waffle with whipped cream and strawberries.

Nutrition:

Carbs: 5 g ;Fat: 14 g ;Protein: 12 g ;Calories: 218

Cream Cheese & Butter Chaffles

Servings: 4

Cooking Time:

16 Minutes

Ingredients:

- 2 tablespoons butter, melted and cooled
- 2 large organic eggs
- 2 ounces cream cheese, softened
- ¼ cup powdered Erythritol
- 1½ teaspoons organic vanilla extract
- Pinch of salt
- ¼ cup almond flour
- 2 tablespoons coconut flour
- 1 teaspoon organic baking powder

Directions:

1. Preheat a mini waffle iron and then grease it.
2. In a bowl, place the butter and eggs and beat until creamy.
3. Add the cream cheese, Erythritol, vanilla extract and salt and beat until well combined.
4. Add the flours and baking powder and beat until well combined.
5. Place ¼ of the mixture into preheated waffle iron and cook for about 4 minutes or until golden brown.
6. Repeat with the remaining mixture.
7. Serve warm.

Nutrition:

Calories: 202 Net Carb: 2 Fat: 17.3 g Saturated Fat: 8 g Carbohydrates: 5.1 g Dietary Fiber: 2.3 g Sugar: 0.7 g Protein: 4.8 g

Chocolate Cherry Chaffles

Servings: 1

Cooking Time:

5 Minutes

Ingredients:

- 1 Tbsp almond flour
- 1 Tbsp cocoa powder
- 1 Tbsp sugar free sweetener
- ½ tsp baking powder
- 1 whole egg
- ½ cup mozzarella cheese shredded
- 2 Tbsp heavy whipping cream whipped
- 2 Tbsp sugar free cherry pie filling
- 1 Tbsp chocolate chips

Directions:

1. Turn on waffle maker to heat and oil it with cooking spray.
2. Mix all dry components in a bowl.
3. Add egg and mix well.
4. Add cheese and stir again.
5. Spoon batter into waffle maker and close.
6. Cook for 5 minutes, until done.
7. Top with whipping cream, cherries, and chocolate chips.

Nutrition:

Carbs: 6 g ;Fat: 1 g ;Protein: 1 g ;Calories: 130

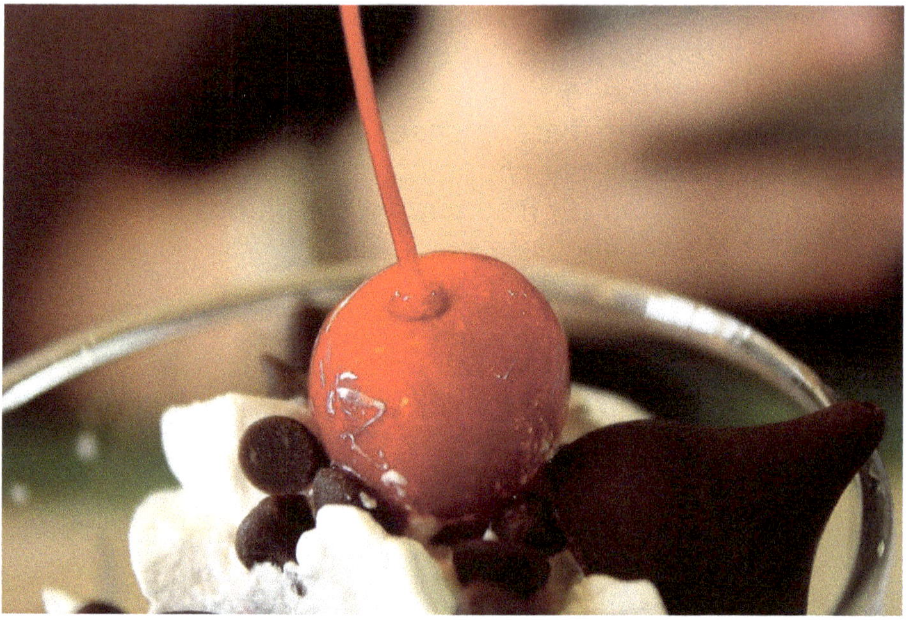

Coconut & Walnut Chaffles

Servings: 8

Cooking Time:

24 Minutes

Ingredients:

- 4 organic eggs, beaten
- 4 ounces cream cheese, softened
- 1 tablespoon butter, melted
- 4 tablespoons coconut flour
- 1 tablespoon almond flour
- 2 tablespoons Erythritol
- 1½ teaspoons organic baking powder
- 1 teaspoon organic vanilla extract
- ½ teaspoon ground cinnamon
- 1 tablespoon unsweetened coconut, shredded
- 1 tablespoon walnuts, chopped

Directions:

1. Preheat a mini waffle iron and then grease it.
2. In a blender, place all ingredients and pulse until creamy and smooth.
3. Divide the mixture into 8 portions.
4. Place 1 portion of the mixture into preheated waffle iron and cook for about 2-3 minutes or until golden brown.
5. Repeat with the remaining mixture.
6. Serve warm.

Nutrition:

Calories: 125 Net Carb: 2.2 g Fat: 10.2 g Saturated Fat: 5.2 g Carbohydrates: 4 g Dietary Fiber: 1.8 g Sugar: 0.4 g Protein: 4.6 g

Chocolate Chaffles

Servings: 2

Cooking Time:

10 Minutes

Ingredients:

- ¾ cup shredded mozzarella
- 1 large egg
- 2 Tbsp almond flour
- 2 Tbsp allulose
- ½ Tbsp melted butter
- 1½ Tbsp cocoa powder
- ½ tsp vanilla extract
- ½ tsp psyllium husk powder
- ¼ tsp baking powder

Directions:

1. Turn on waffle maker to heat and oil it with cooking spray.
2. Mix all ingredients in a small bowl.
3. Pour ¼ cup batter into a 4-inch waffle maker.
4. Cook for 2-3 minutes, or until crispy.
5. Transfer chaffle to a plate and set aside.
6. Repeat with remaining batter.

Nutrition:

Carbs: 6 g ;Fat: 24 g ;Protein: 15 g ;Calories: 296

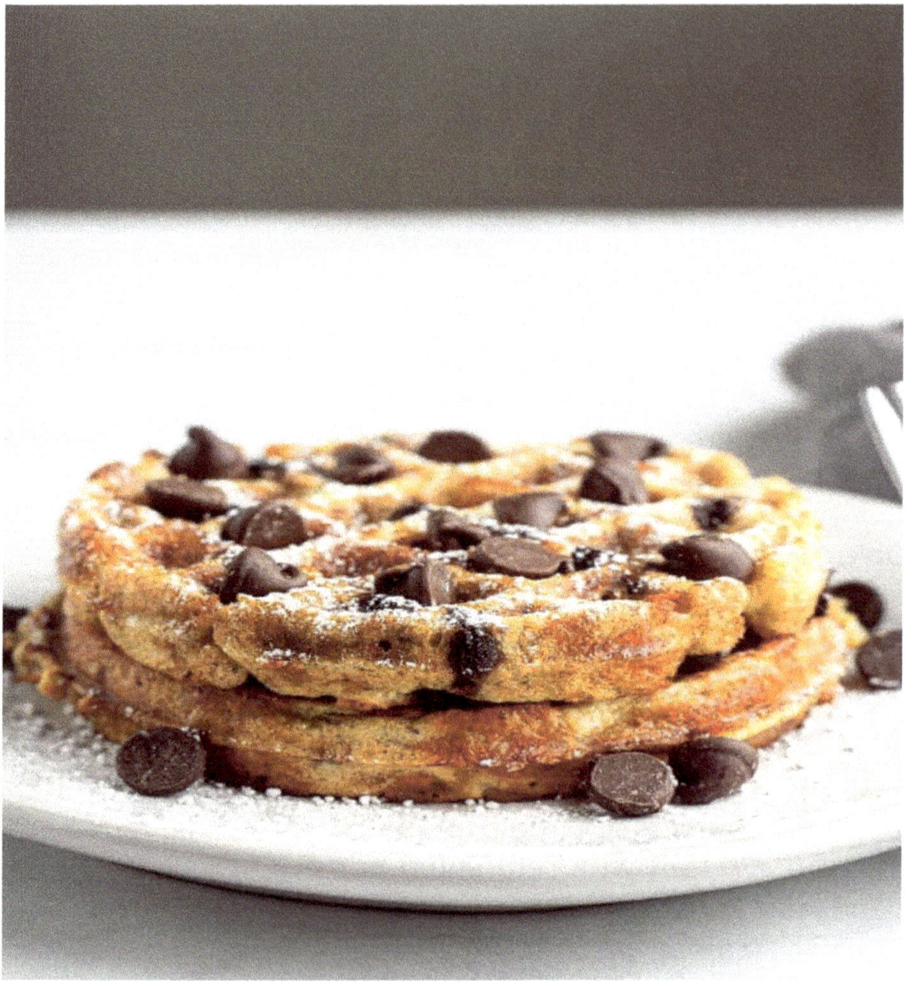

Chocolate Chips & Whipping Cream Chaffles

Servings: 2

Cooking Time:

8 Minutes

Ingredients:

- 1 organic egg
- 1 tablespoon heavy whipping cream
- ½ teaspoon coconut flour
- 1¾ teaspoons monkfruit sweetener
- ¼ teaspoon organic baking powder
- Pinch of salt
- 1 tablespoon 70% dark chocolate chips

Directions:

1. Preheat a mini waffle iron and then grease it.
2. In a bowl, place all ingredients except for chocolate chips and beat until well combined.
3. Fold in the blackberries.
4. Place half of the mixture into preheated waffle iron and top with half of the chocolate chips.
5. Cook for about 3-4 minutes or until golden brown.
6. Repeat with the remaining mixture and chocolate chips.
7. Serve warm.

Nutrition:

Calories: 110 Net Carb: 1 Fat: 9 g Saturated Fat: 5 g Carbohydrates: 3.1 g Dietary Fiber: 1.3 g Sugar: 0.2 g Protein: 4 g

Spiced Pumpkin Chaffles

Servings: 2

Cooking Time:

8 Minutes

Ingredients:

- 1 organic egg, beaten
- ½ cup Mozzarella cheese, shredded
- 1 tablespoon sugar-free canned solid pumpkin
- ¼ teaspoon ground cinnamon
- Pinch of ground cloves
- Pinch of ground nutmeg
- Pinch of ground ginger

Directions:

1. Preheat a mini waffle iron and then grease it.
2. In a medium bowl, place all ingredients and with a fork, mix until well combined.
3. Place half of the mixture into preheated waffle iron and cook for about 4 minutes or until golden brown.
4. Repeat with the remaining mixture.
5. Serve warm.

Nutrition:

Calories: 5 Carb: 1 g Fat: 3.5 g Saturated Fat: 1.5 g Carbohydrates: 1.4 g Dietary Fiber: 0.4 g Sugar: 0.5 g Protein: 4.9 g

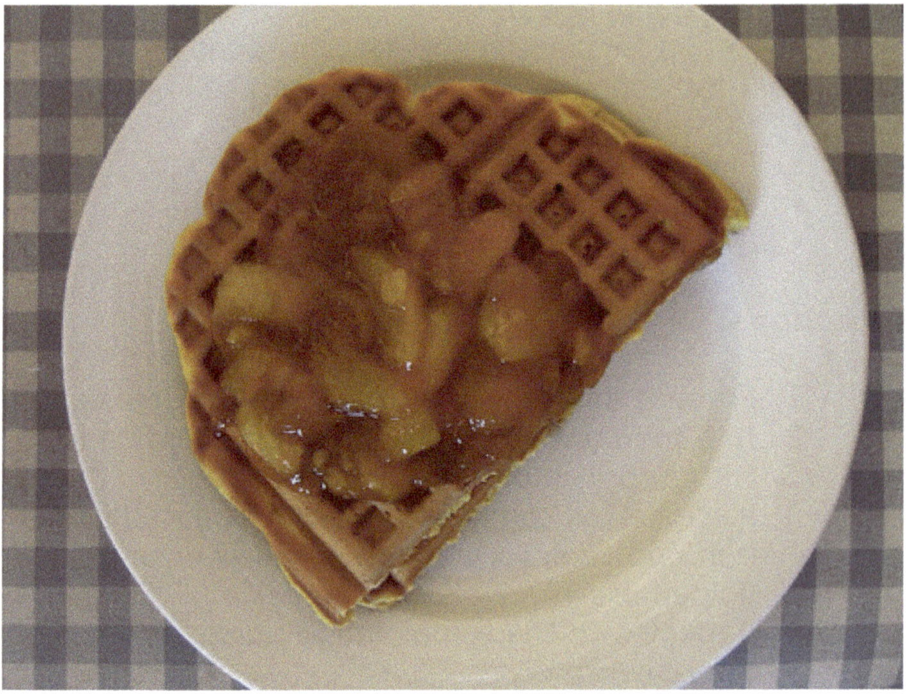

Vanilla Chaffle

Servings: 2

Cooking Time:

8 Minutes

Ingredients:

- 2 tbsp butter, softened
- 2 oz cream cheese, softened
- 2 eggs
- ¼ cup almond flour
- 2 tbsp coconut flour
- 1 tsp baking powder
- 1 tsp vanilla extract
- ¼ cup confectioners
- Pinch of pink salt

Directions:

1. Preheat the waffle maker and spray with non-stick cooking spray.
2. Melt the butter and set aside for a minute to cool.
3. Add the eggs into the melted butter and whisk until creamy.
4. Pour in the sweetener, vanilla, extract, and salt. Blend properly.
5. Next add the coconut flour, almond flour, and baking powder. Mix well.
6. Pour into the waffle maker and cook for 4 minutes.
7. Repeat the process with the remaining batter.
8. Remove and set aside to cool.
9. Enjoy.

Nutrition:

Calories per Servings: 202 Kcal ; Fats: 27 g ; Carbs: 9 g ; Protein: 23 g

Banana Nut Chaffle

Servings: 1

Cooking Time:

10 Minutes

Ingredients:

- 1 egg
- 1 Tbsp cream cheese, softened and room temp
- 1 Tbsp sugar-free cheesecake pudding
- ½ cup mozzarella cheese
- 1 Tbsp monk fruit confectioners sweetener
- ¼ tsp vanilla extract
- ¼ tsp banana extract
- toppings of choice

Directions:

1. Turn on waffle maker to heat and oil it with cooking spray.
2. Beat egg in a small bowl.
3. Add remaining ingredients and mix until well incorporated.
4. Add one half of the batter to waffle maker and cook for minutes, until golden brown.
5. Remove chaffle and add the other half of the batter.
6. Top with your optional toppings and serve warm!

Nutrition:

Carbs: 2 g ;Fat: g ;Protein: 8 g ;Calories: 119

Chocolaty Chips Pumpkin Chaffles

Servings: 3

Cooking Time:

12 Minutes

Ingredients:

- 1 organic egg
- 4 teaspoons homemade pumpkin puree
- ½ cup Mozzarella cheese, shredded
- 1 tablespoon almond flour
- 2 tablespoons granulated Erythritol
- ¼ teaspoon pumpkin pie spice
- 4 teaspoons 70% dark chocolate chips

Directions:

1. In a bowl, place the egg and pumpkin puree and mix well.
2. Add the remaining ingredients except for chocolate chips and mix until well combined.
3. Gently, fold in the chocolate chips and lemon zest.
4. Place 1/3 of the mixture into preheated waffle iron and cook for about minutes or until golden brown.
5. Repeat with the remaining mixture.
6. Serve warm.

Nutrition:

Calories: 9 Carb: 1.9 g Fat: 7.1 g Saturated Fat: 3.3 g Carbohydrates: 1.4 g Dietary Fiber: 2.6 g Sugar: 0.4 g Protein: 4.2 g

Oreo Chaffles

Servings: 2

Cooking Time:

5 Minutes

Ingredients:

- Chocolate Chaffle:
- 2 eggs
- 2 tbsp cocoa, unsweetened
- 2 tbsp sweetener
- 2 tbsp heavy cream
- 2 tsp coconut flour
- 1/2 tsp baking powder
- 1 tsp vanilla
- Filling:
- Whipped cream

Directions:

- Pour half of the mixture into the waffle iron. Cook for 5 minutes.
- Once ready, carefully remove and repeat with the remaining chaffle mixture.
- Allow the cooked chaffles to sit for 3 minutes.
- Once they have cooled, spread the whipped cream on the chaffles and stack them cream side facing down to form a sandwich.
- Slice into halves and enjoy.

Nutrition:

Calories per Servings: 390 Kcal ; Fats: 40 g ; Carbs: 3 g ; Protein: 10 g

Whipping Cream Pumpkin Chaffles

Servings: 4

Cooking Time:

12 Minutes

Ingredients:

- 2 organic eggs
- 2 tablespoons homemade pumpkin puree
- 2 tablespoons heavy whipping cream
- 1 tablespoon coconut flour
- 1 tablespoon Erythritol
- 1 teaspoon pumpkin pie spice
- ½ teaspoon organic baking powder
- ½ teaspoon organic vanilla extract
- Pinch of salt
- ½ cup Mozzarella cheese, shredded

Directions:

1. Preheat a mini waffle iron and then grease it.
2. In a bowl, place all the ingredients except Mozzarella cheese and beat until well combined.
3. Add the Mozzarella cheese and stir to combine.
4. Place half of the mixture into preheated waffle iron and cook for about 6 minutes or until golden brown.
5. Repeat with the remaining mixture.
6. Serve warm.

Nutrition:

Calories: 81 Net Carb: 2.1 g Fat: 5.9 g Saturated Fat: 3 g Carbohydrates: 3.1 g Dietary Fiber: 1 g Sugar: 0.5 g Protein: 4.3 g

Chocolate Vanilla Chaffles

Servings: 2

Cooking Time:

5 Minutes

Ingredients:

- ½ cup shredded mozzarella cheese
- 1 egg
- 1 Tbsp granulated sweetener
- 1 tsp vanilla extract
- 1 Tbsp sugar-free chocolate chips
- 2 Tbsp almond meal/flour

Directions:

1. Turn on waffle maker to heat and oil it with cooking spray.
2. Mix all components in a bowl until combined.
3. Pour half of the batter into waffle maker.
4. Cook for 2-minutes, then remove and repeat with remaining batter.
5. Top with more chips and favorite toppings.

Nutrition:

Carbs: 23 g ;Fat: 3 g ;Protein: 4 g ;Calories: 134

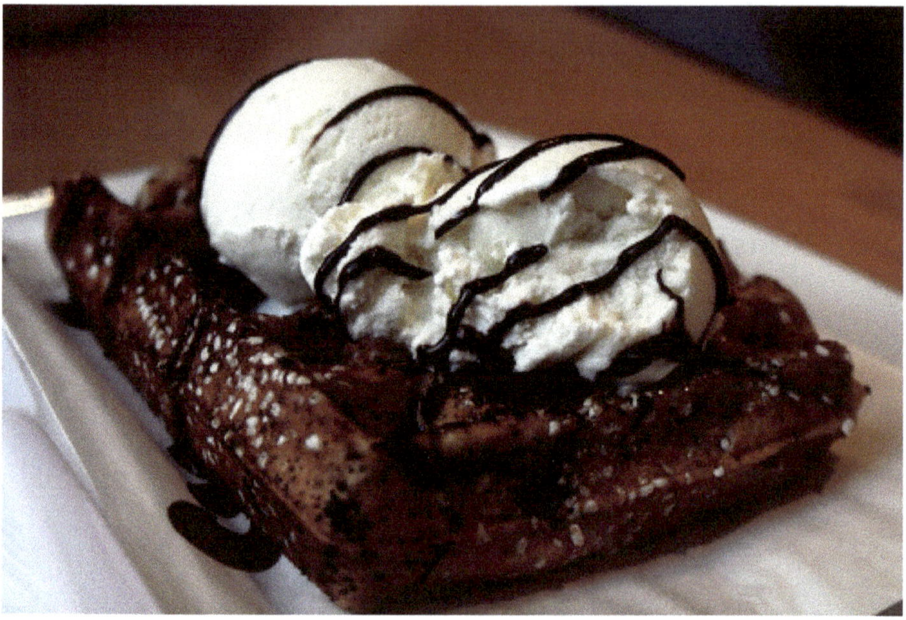

Churro Waffles

Servings: 1

Cooking Time:

10 Minutes

Ingredients:

- 1 tbsp coconut cream
- 1 egg
- 6 tbsp almond flour
- ¼ tsp xanthan gum
- ½ tsp cinnamon
- 2 tbsp keto brown sugar
- Coating:
- 2 tbsp butter, melt
- 1 tbsp keto brown sugar
- Warm up your waffle maker.

Directions:

- Pour half of the batter to the waffle pan and cook for 5 minutes.
- Carefully remove the cooked waffle and repeat the steps with the remaining batter.
- Allow the chaffles to cool and spread with the melted butter and top with the brown sugar.
- Enjoy.

Nutrition:

Calories per Servings: 178 Kcal ; Fats: 15.7 g ; Carbs: 3.9 g ; Protein: 2 g

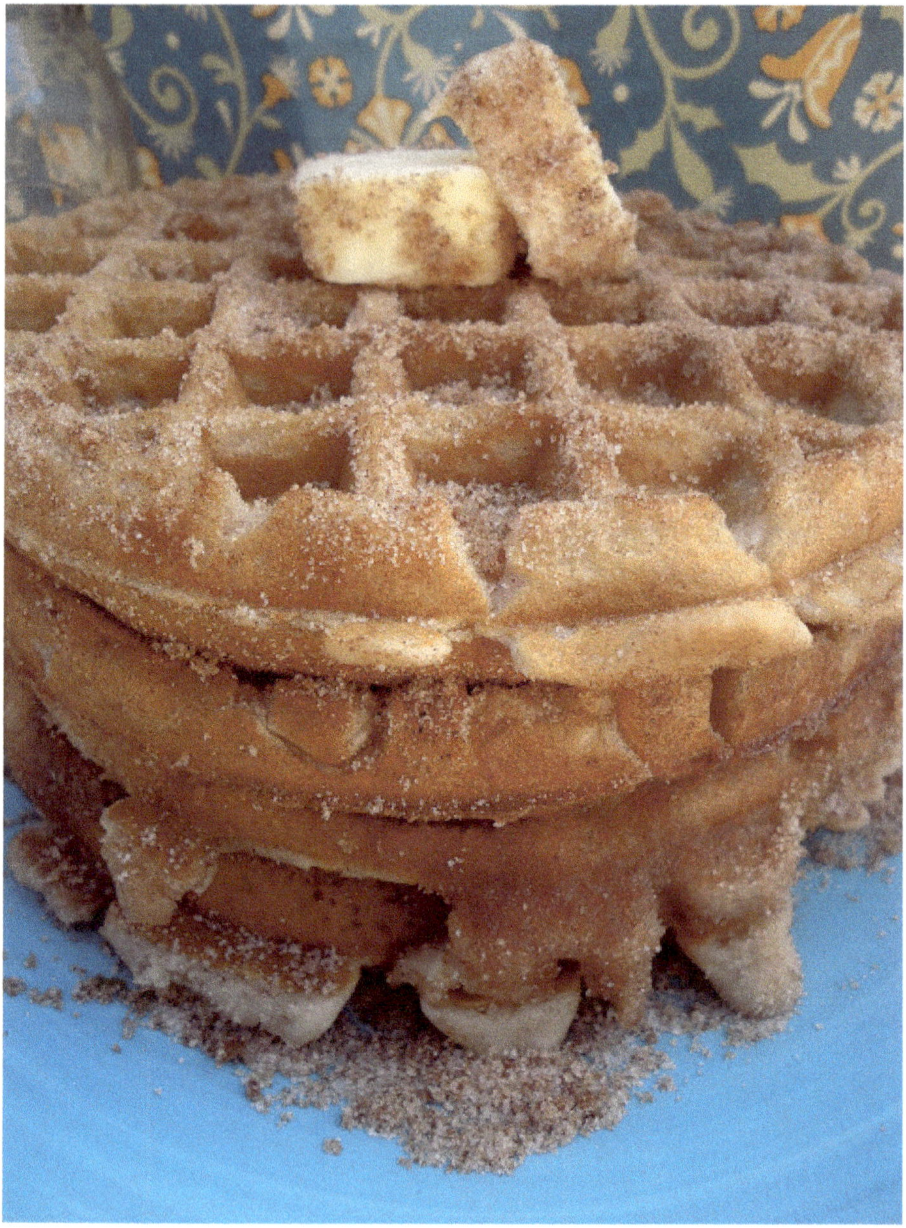

Chocolate Chips Lemon Chaffles

Servings: 4

Cooking Time:

8 Minutes

Ingredients:

- 2 organic eggs
- ½ cup Mozzarella cheese, shredded
- ¾ teaspoon organic lemon extract
- ½ teaspoon organic vanilla extract
- 2 teaspoons Erythritol
- ½ teaspoon psyllium husk powder
- Pinch of salt
- 1 tablespoon 70% dark chocolate chips
- ¼ teaspoon lemon zest, grated finely

Directions:

1. Preheat a mini waffle iron and then grease it.
2. In a bowl, place all ingredients except chocolate chips and lemon zest and beat until well combined.
3. Gently, fold in the chocolate chips and lemon zest.
4. Place ¼ of the mixture into preheated waffle iron and cook for about minutes or until golden brown.
5. Repeat with the remaining mixture.
6. Serve warm.

Nutrition:

Calories: Net Carb: 1 g Fat: 4.8 g Saturated Fat: 2.3 g Carbohydrates: 1.5 g Dietary Fiber: 0.5 g Sugar: 0.3 g Protein: 4.3 g

Mocha Chaffles

Servings: 3

Cooking Time:

9 Minutes

Ingredients:

- 1 organic egg, beaten
- 1 tablespoon cacao powder
- 1 tablespoon Erythritol
- ¼ teaspoon organic baking powder
- 2 tablespoons cream cheese, softened
- 1 tablespoon mayonnaise
- ¼ teaspoon instant coffee powder
- Pinch of salt
- 1 teaspoon organic vanilla extract

Directions:

1. Preheat a mini waffle iron and then grease it.
2. In a medium bowl, place all ingredients and with a fork, mix until well combined.
3. Place 1/of the mixture into preheated waffle iron and cook for about 2½-3 minutes or until golden brown.
4. Repeat with the remaining mixture.
5. Serve warm.

Nutrition:

Calories: 83 Net Carb: 1 g Fat: 7.5 g Saturated Fat: 4 Carbohydrates: 1.5 g Dietary Fiber: 0.5 g Sugar: 0.3 g Protein: 2.7 g

Carrot Chaffles

Servings: 6

Cooking Time:

18 Minutes

Ingredients:

- ¾ cup almond flour
- 1 tablespoon walnuts, chopped
- 2 tablespoons powdered Erythritol
- 1 teaspoon organic baking powder
- ½ teaspoon ground cinnamon
- ½ teaspoon pumpkin pie spice
- 1 organic egg, beaten
- 2 tablespoons heavy whipping cream
- 2 tablespoons butter, melted
- ½ cup carrot, peeled and shredded

Directions:

1. Preheat a mini waffle iron and then grease it.
2. In a bowl, place the flour, walnut, Erythritol, cinnamon, baking powder and spices and mix well.
3. Add the egg, heavy whipping cream and butter and mix until well combined.
4. Gently, fold in the carrot.
5. Add about 3 tablespoons of the mixture into preheated waffle iron and cook for about 2½-3 minutes or until golden brown.
6. Repeat with the remaining mixture.
7. Serve warm.

Nutrition:

Calories: 165 Net Carb: 2.4 g Fat: 14.7 g Saturated Fat: 4.4 g Carbohydrates: 4.4 g Dietary Fiber: 2 g Sugar: 1 g Protein: 1.5 g

Yogurt Chaffles

Servings: 3

Cooking Time:

10 Minutes

Ingredients:

- ½ cup shredded mozzarella
- 1 egg
- 2 Tbsp ground almonds
- ½ tsp psyllium husk
- ¼ tsp baking powder
- 1 Tbsp yogurt

Directions:

1. Turn on waffle maker to heat and oil it with cooking spray.
2. Whisk eggs in a bowl.
3. Add in remaining ingredients except mozzarella and mix well.
4. Add mozzarella and mix once again. Let it sit for 5 minutes.
5. Add ⅓ cup batter into each waffle mold.
6. Close and cook for 4-5 minutes.
7. Repeat with remaining batter.

Nutrition:

Carbs: 2 g ;Fat: 5 g ;Protein: 4 g ;Calories: 93

Chocolate Peanut Butter Chaffles

Servings: 2

Cooking Time:

8 Minutes

Ingredients:

- 1 organic egg, beaten
- ¼ cup mozzarella cheese, shredded
- 2 tablespoons creamy peanut butter
- 1 tablespoon almond flour
- 1 tablespoon granulated erythritol
- 1 teaspoon organic vanilla extract
- 1 tablespoon 70% dark chocolate chips

Directions:

1. Preheat a mini waffle iron and then grease it.
2. In a bowl, add all ingredients except chocolate and beat until well combined.
3. Gently, fold in the chocolate chips.
4. Place half of the mixture into preheated waffle iron and cook for about 4 minutes.
5. Repeat with the remaining mixture.
6. Serve warm.

Nutrition:

Calories 214 Net Carbs 4.1 g Total Fat 18 g Saturated Fat 5.4 g Cholesterol 84 mg Sodium 128 mg Total Carbs 6.4 g Fiber 2.3 g Sugar 2.1 g Protein 8.8 g

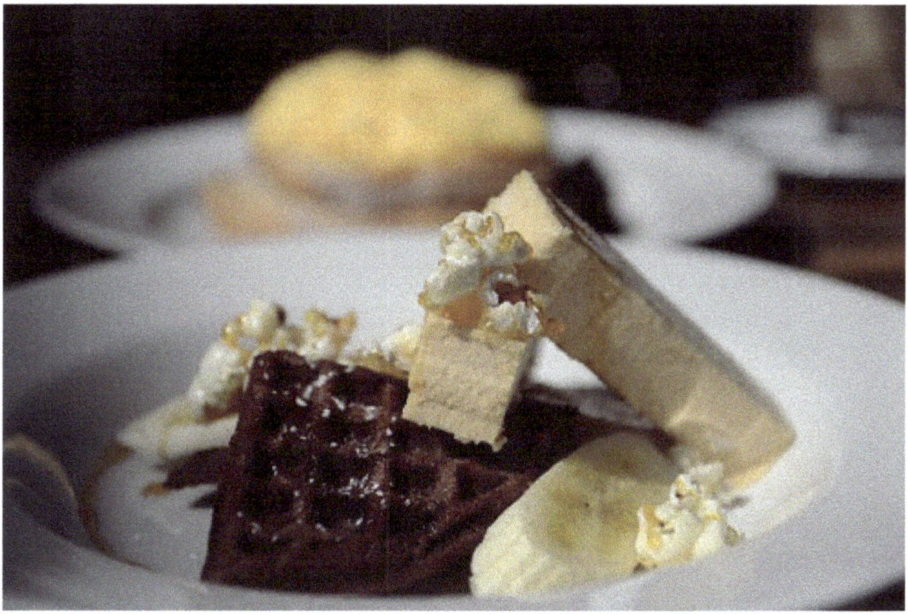

Ube Chaffles With Ice Cream

Servings: 2

Cooking Time:

10 Minutes

Ingredients:

- 1/3 cup mozzarella cheese, shredded
- 1 tbsp whipped cream cheese
- 2 tbsp sweetener
- 1 egg
- 2-3 drops ube or pandan extract
- 1/2 tsp baking powder
- Keto ice cream

Directions:

1. Add in 2 or 3 drops of ube extract, mix until creamy and smooth.
2. Pour half of the batter mixture in the mini waffle maker and cook for about 5 minutes.
3. Repeat the same steps with the remaining batter mixture.
4. Top with keto ice cream and enjoy.
5. Note: more keto stuffing you can find in my easy desserts cookbook here:

Nutrition:

Calories per Servings: 265Kca l ; Fats: 16 g ; Carbs: 7 g ; Protein: 22 g

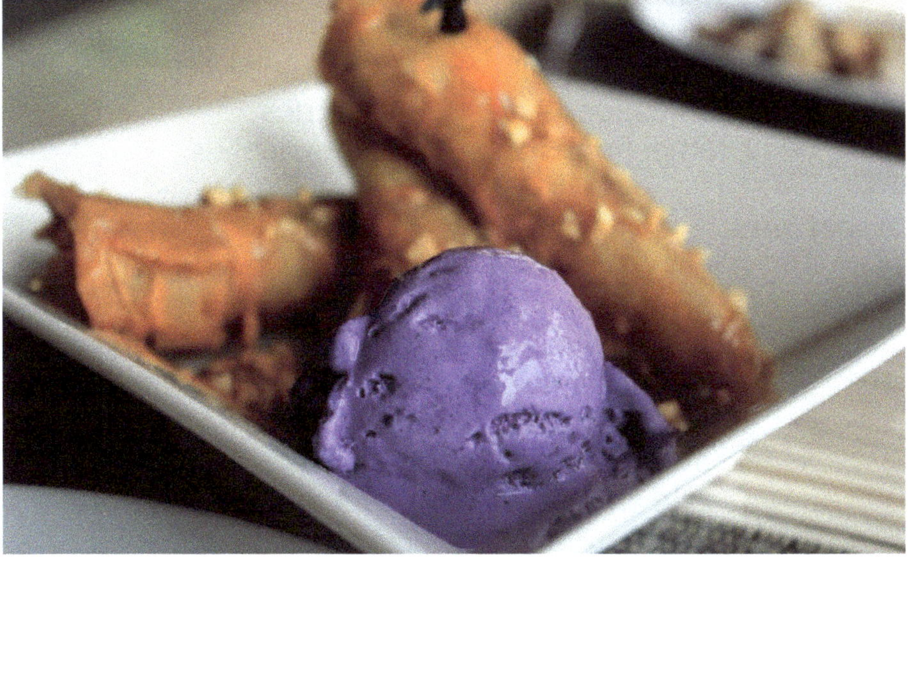

2- Berries Chaffles

Servings: 2

Cooking Time:

10 Minutes

Ingredients:

- 1 organic egg
- 1 teaspoon organic vanilla extract
- 1 tablespoon of almond flour
- 1 teaspoon organic baking powder
- Pinch of ground cinnamon
- 1 cup Mozzarella cheese, shredded
- 2 tablespoons fresh blueberries
- 2 tablespoons fresh blackberries

Directions:

1. Preheat a waffle iron and then grease it.
2. In a bowl, place thee egg and vanilla extract and beat well.
3. Add the flour, baking powder and cinnamon and mix well.
4. Add the Mozzarella cheese and mix until just combined.
5. Gently, fold in the berries.
6. Place half of the mixture into preheated waffle iron and cook for about 4-5 minutes or until golden brown.
7. Repeat with the remaining mixture.
8. Serve warm.

Nutrition:

Calories: 112 Net Carb: 3.8 g Fat: 6.7 g Saturated Fat: 2.3 g Carbohydrates: 5 g Dietary Fiber: 1.2 g Sugar: 1 Protein: 7 g

Cinnamon Swirl Chaffles

Servings: 3

Cooking Time:

12 Minutes

Ingredients:

- For Chaffles:
- 1 organic egg
- ½ cup Mozzarella cheese, shredded
- 1 tablespoon almond flour
- ¼ teaspoon organic baking powder
- 1 teaspoon granulated Erythritol
- 1 teaspoon ground cinnamon
- For Topping:
- 1 tablespoon butter
- 1 teaspoon ground cinnamon
- 2 teaspoons powdered Erythritol

Directions:

1. Preheat a waffle iron and then grease it.
2. For chaffles: in a bowl, place all ingredients and mix until well combined.
3. For topping: in a small microwave-safe bowl, place all ingredients and microwave for about 15 seconds.
4. Remove from microwave and mix well.
5. Place 1/3 of the chaffles mixture into preheated waffle iron.
6. Top with 1/3 of the butter mixture and with a skewer, gently swirl into the chaffles mixture.
7. Cook for about 3-4 minutes or until golden brown.

8. Repeat with the remaining chaffles and topping mixture.
9. Serve warm.

Nutrition:

Calories: 87 Net Carb: 1 g Fat: 7.4 g Saturated Fat: 3.5 g Carbohydrates: 2.1 g Dietary Fiber: 1.1 g Sugar: 0.2 g Protein: 3.3 g

Chocolate Cream Cheese Chaffles

Servings: 2

Cooking Time:

8 Minutes

Ingredients:

- 1 large organic egg, beaten
- 1 ounce cream cheese, softened
- 1 tablespoon sugar-free chocolate syrup
- 1 tablespoon Erythritol
- ½ tablespoon cacao powder
- ¼ teaspoon organic baking powder
- ½ teaspoon organic vanilla extract

Directions:

1. Preheat a mini waffle iron and then grease it.
2. In a medium bowl, place all ingredients and with a fork, mix until well combined.
3. Place half of the mixture into preheated waffle iron and cook for about 4 minutes or until golden brown.
4. Repeat with the remaining mixture.
5. Serve warm.

Nutrition:

Calories: 103 Net Carb: 4.2 g Fat: 7.7 g Saturated Fat: 4.1 g Carbohydrates: 4 Dietary Fiber: 0.4 g Sugar: 2 g Protein: 4.5 g

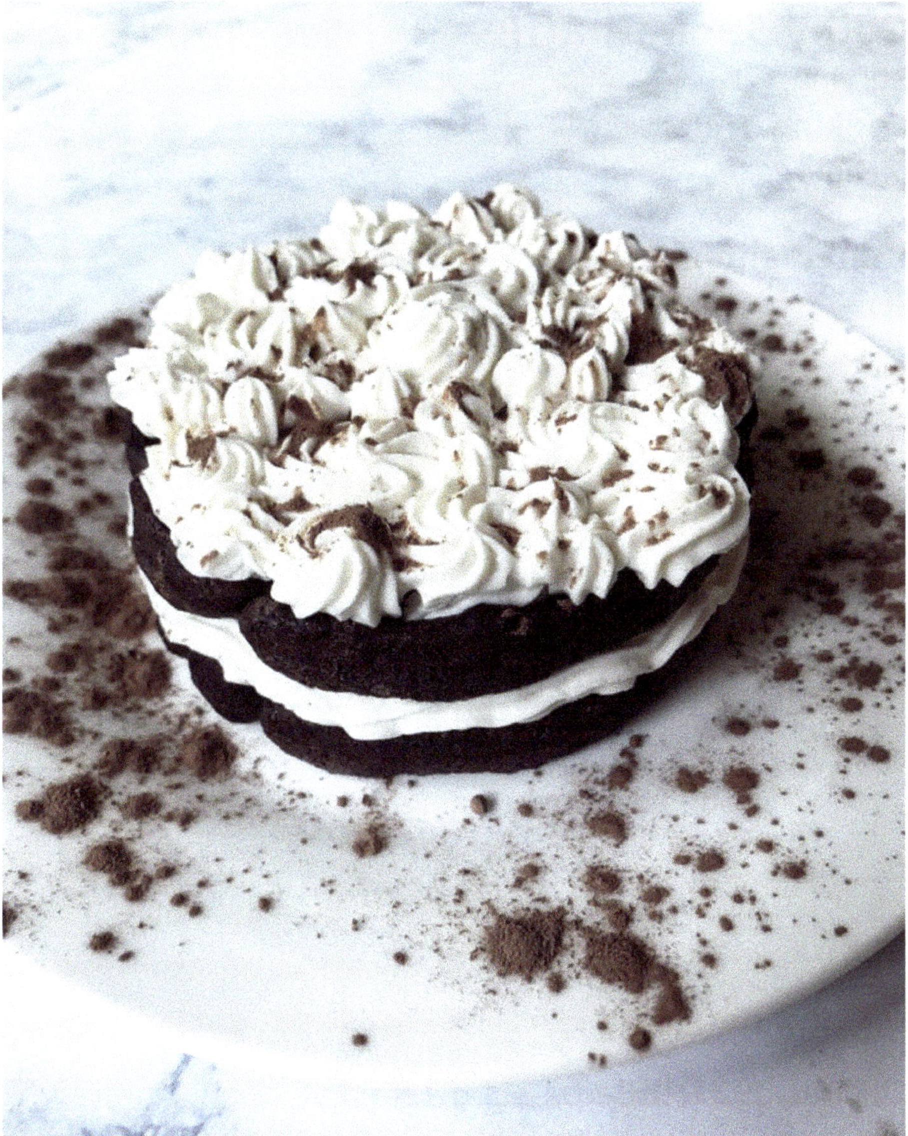

Colby Jack Chaffles

Servings: 1

Cooking Time:

6 Minutes

Ingredients:

- 2 ounces colby jack cheese, sliced thinly in triangles
- 1 large organic egg, beaten

Directions:

1. Preheat a waffle iron and then grease it.
2. Arrange 1 thin layer of cheese slices in the bottom of preheated waffle iron.
3. Place the beaten egg on top of the cheese.
4. Now, arrange another layer of cheese slices on top to cover evenly.
5. Cook for about 6 minutes.
6. Serve warm.

Nutrition:

Calories 292 Net Carbs 2.4 g Total Fat 23 g Saturated Fat 13.6 g Cholesterol 236 mg Sodium 431 mg Total Carbs 2.4 g Fiber 0 g Sugar 0.4 g Protein 18.3 g

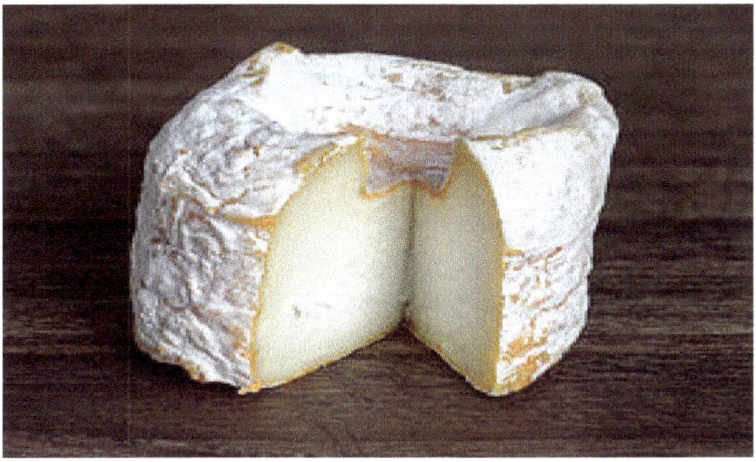

Chaffle Birthday Cake

Servings: 4

Cooking Time:

16 Minutes

Ingredients:

- Butter cream icing
- Birthday Cake Chaffle:
- 3 tbsp cream cheese
- 1 tbsp almond flour
- 5 tbsp coconut flour
- 1 tsp baking powder
- 6 eggs
- 2 tbsp birthday cake syrup

Directions:

1. Scoop 3 tbsp of the mixture into your waffle maker. Cook for 4 minutes and set aside.
2. Repeat the process until you have 4 cake chaffles.
3. Just like a normal cake, start assembling your cake by placing one chaffle at the bottom as the base and add a butter cream icing layer.
4. Repeat the same process.
5. Pipe your cake edges with the icing and pile colorful shredded coconut at the centre.
6. Once all the layers are completed, top with more icing and shredded coconut sprinkles.
7. Enjoy!

Nutrition:

Calories: 390 Kcal ; Fats: 35 g ; Carbs: 18.9 g ; Protein: 11 g

Chaffle Churros

Servings: 2

Cooking Time:

5 Minutes

Ingredients:

- 1 egg
- 1 Tbsp almond flour
- ½ tsp vanilla extract
- 1 tsp cinnamon, divided
- ¼ tsp baking powder
- ½ cup shredded mozzarella
- 1 Tbsp swerve confectioners sugar substitute
- 1 Tbsp swerve brown sugar substitute
- 1 Tbsp butter, melted

Directions:

1. Turn on waffle maker to heat and oil it with cooking spray.
2. Mix egg, flour, vanilla extract, ½ tsp cinnamon, baking powder, mozzarella, and sugar substitute in a bowl.
3. Place half of the mixture into waffle maker and cook for 5 minutes, or until desired doneness.
4. Remove and place the second half of the batter into the maker.
5. Cut chaffles into strips.
6. Place strips in a bowl and cover with melted butter.
7. Mix brown sugar substitute and the remaining cinnamon in a bowl.
8. Pour sugar mixture over the strips and toss to coat them well.

Nutrition:

Carbs: 5 g ; Fat: 6 g ;Protein: 5 g ;Calories: 76

Strawberry Chaffles

Servings: 2

Cooking Time:

8 Minutes

Ingredients:

- 1 organic egg, beaten
- ¼ cup Mozzarella cheese, shredded
- 1 tablespoon cream cheese, softened
- ¼ teaspoon organic baking powder
- 1 teaspoon organic strawberry extract
- 2 fresh strawberries, hulled and sliced

Directions:

1. Preheat a mini waffle iron and then grease it.
2. In a bowl, place all ingredients except strawberry slices and beat until well combined.
3. Fold in the strawberry slices.
4. Place half of the mixture into preheated waffle iron and cook for about minutes or until golden brown.
5. Repeat with the remaining mixture.
6. Serve warm.

Nutrition:

Calories: 69 Net Carb: 1.6 g Fat: 4.6 g Saturated Fat: 2.2 g Carbohydrates: 1.9 g Dietary Fiber: 0.3 g Sugar: 1 g Protein: 4.2 g

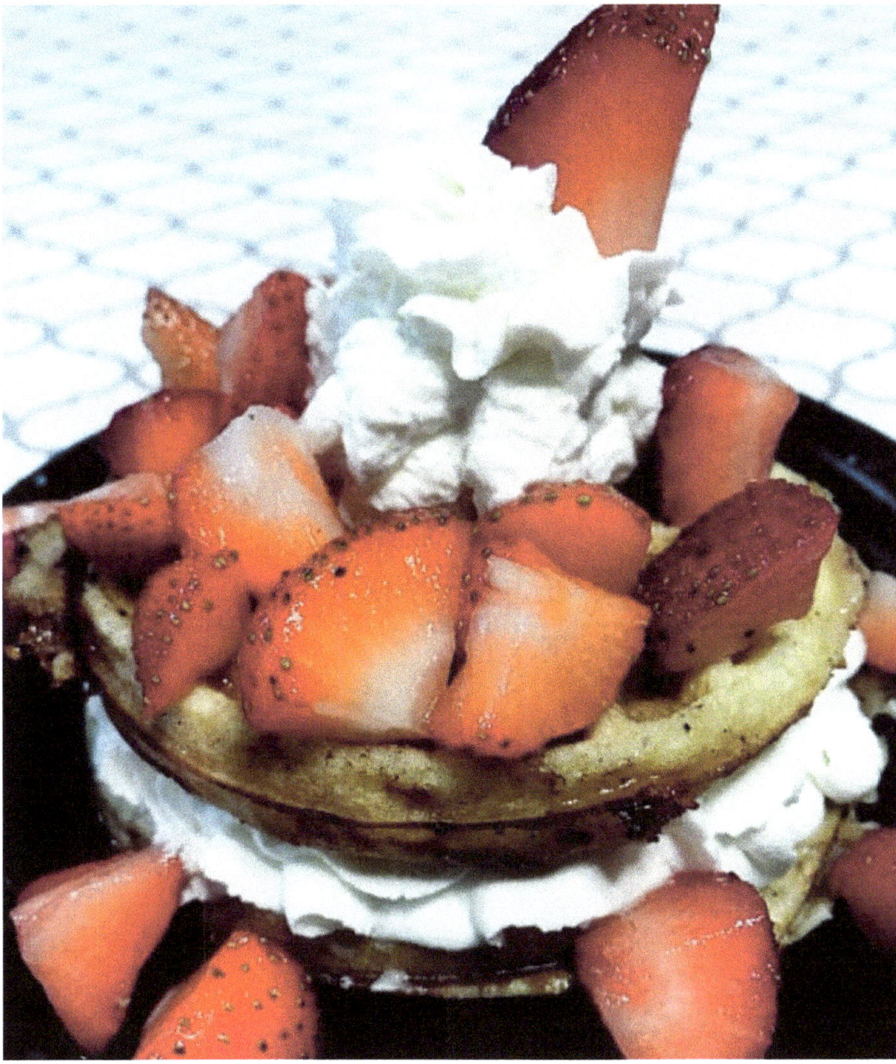

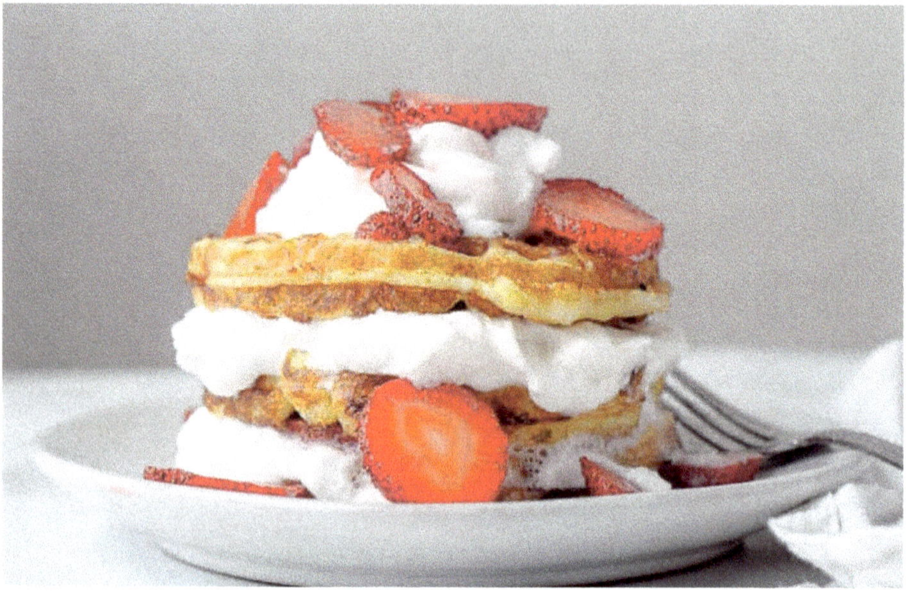

Lightning Source UK Ltd.
Milton Keynes UK
UKHW020641210621
385885UK00001B/58

9 781803 177687